Mastering Epic: A Comprehensive Guide to Electronic Health Records (EHR) and Practice Management (PM)

Glossary of Epic Terminology

Useful Resources for Epic Users

Index

This comprehensive book, "Mastering Epic: A Comprehensive Guide to Electronic Health Records (EHR) and Practice Management (PM)," will provide healthcare professionals, administrators, and IT professionals with a deep understanding of Epic's capabilities, its role in improving healthcare delivery, and practical guidance for effective implementation and utilization. Each chapter covers essential topics related to Epic, making it a valuable resource for anyone looking to maximize the benefits of this powerful electronic health records and practice management system.

Table of Contents

Chapter 1: Introduction to Epic

In this chapter, we'll start your journey into the world of Epic, the leading Electronic Health Records (EHR) and Practice Management (PM) system in healthcare. By the end of this tutorial, you'll have a solid grasp of what Epic is, its significance in healthcare, and the historical context that has shaped its evolution.

Section 1: Understanding the Role of Epic in Healthcare

1.1 What is Epic?

Epic is a comprehensive and integrated EHR and PM software system used by healthcare organizations around the world. It serves as a digital repository for patient information, streamlines clinical workflows, and assists in practice management tasks. Essentially, it's the backbone of modern healthcare operations, enhancing patient care and optimizing healthcare delivery.

1.2 The Importance of EHR and PM

Electronic Health Records (EHR) and Practice Management (PM) systems like Epic have revolutionized the healthcare industry. They offer several key benefits:
Improved Patient Care: EHRs provide quick access to patient records, reducing errors and enabling healthcare providers to make informed decisions.

Efficiency: PM systems streamline administrative tasks such as scheduling, billing, and claims management, freeing up more time for patient care.

Interoperability: Epic facilitates the exchange of patient data between healthcare providers, promoting better coordination of care.

Data Analytics: Epic's robust reporting and analytics tools enable healthcare organizations to derive insights from patient data, leading to more informed decisions and improved outcomes.

1.3 Why Epic?

Epic has become synonymous with quality and reliability in the healthcare industry for several reasons:

Comprehensive Solutions: Epic offers a wide range of modules and applications, covering virtually every aspect of healthcare, from clinical documentation to billing.

Customization: Organizations can tailor Epic to meet their specific needs, ensuring a personalized and efficient workflow.

Scalability: Epic scales to accommodate healthcare organizations of all sizes, from small practices to large hospital systems.

Section 2: Evolution and History of Epic Systems

1.4 The Birth of Epic
Epic Systems Corporation was founded in 1979 by Judy

Faulkner in Madison, Wisconsin. It initially started as a small software consulting firm, and its first product, the EpicCare EHR system, was released in the late 1990s. Since then, it has grown exponentially, becoming a leader in the EHR and PM industry.

1.5 Key Milestones

EpicCare: The release of Epic's first EHR system marked a significant step in digitizing healthcare records and improving patient care.

Interoperability: Epic played a pivotal role in promoting data exchange standards, contributing to improved interoperability between different healthcare systems.

Meaningful Use: Epic systems played a crucial role in helping healthcare organizations achieve meaningful use requirements, unlocking government incentives for EHR adoption.

1.6 Epic Today

Today, Epic serves thousands of healthcare organizations worldwide. Its software is used in hospitals, clinics, long-term care facilities, and more. It continues to evolve, offering cutting-edge features and innovations to support the ever-changing landscape of healthcare.

In the next chapter, we will delve deeper into Epic's impact on healthcare and explore how it has transformed patient care and administrative processes. You'll also get a glimpse of the practical applications and benefits of using Epic.

Chapter 2: Epic's Impact on Healthcare

In this chapter, we'll dive deeper into how Epic has revolutionized healthcare. We'll explore the tangible benefits it brings to patient care, administrative efficiency, and the overall healthcare ecosystem.

Section 1: Improving Patient Care with Epic

2.1 Enhanced Patient Record Management

One of the most significant contributions of Epic to healthcare is the centralization and digitization of patient records. Here's how it improves patient care:

Accessibility: Epic allows healthcare providers to access patient records from anywhere, providing real-time data at the point of care. This access enables quicker and more informed decision-making.

Data Accuracy: With Epic, patient records are more accurate and complete, reducing the risk of errors due to illegible handwriting or missing information.

Clinical Decision Support: Epic offers clinical decision support tools that help healthcare providers make evidence-based decisions. Alerts and reminders prompt clinicians to follow best practices and adhere to guidelines.
2.2 Coordination of Care
Epic facilitates better coordination of care among different healthcare providers and departments. Here's how:

Interoperability: Epic's interoperability capabilities allow for seamless sharing of patient data with other healthcare systems, ensuring that everyone involved in a patient's care has access to relevant information.

Care Plans: Epic supports the creation and management of care plans, making it easier to coordinate care among different providers and track patient progress.

Section 2: Epic's Contribution to Healthcare Efficiency

2.3 Streamlined Clinical Workflows
Epic helps healthcare organizations streamline clinical workflows in the following ways:

Efficient Charting: Clinicians can use Epic to efficiently document patient encounters, reducing the time spent on paperwork and administrative tasks.
Order Management: Epic's order management system allows for quick and accurate ordering of tests, medications, and procedures, reducing delays and errors.

2.4 Practice Management Efficiency

Epic isn't just about clinical care; it also plays a vital role in practice management:
Appointment Scheduling: With Epic, practices can manage appointments more effectively, reducing scheduling conflicts and improving patient satisfaction.
Billing and Revenue Cycle Management: Epic's billing and revenue cycle management tools help practices maximize revenue by ensuring accurate and timely claims submission.

Section 3: Real-world Examples

2.5 Case Studies

Let's look at a couple of real-world examples to illustrate the impact of Epic on healthcare:

Hospital A: After implementing Epic, Hospital A reduced medication errors by 30% and saw a 20% increase in patient satisfaction scores.

Medical Practice B: Medical Practice B reported a 40% reduction in administrative overhead after adopting Epic for practice management tasks.

Section 4: Learning from Epic's Impact

2.6 Embracing Epic's Benefits

As a healthcare professional or administrator, understanding Epic's impact is crucial. Here are some key takeaways:

Improved Patient Outcomes: Epic contributes to better patient care by providing timely and accurate information to healthcare providers.

Operational Efficiency: By streamlining workflows and automating administrative tasks, Epic helps healthcare organizations operate more efficiently.

Data-Driven Decision Making: The data collected in Epic can be analyzed to identify trends, measure performance, and inform strategic decisions.

In the next chapter, we'll dive into the Epic user interface, helping you become comfortable with navigating the system and customizing it to your needs. You'll be well on your way to mastering Epic's capabilities.

Chapter 3: Navigating the Epic Interface

In this chapter, we'll guide you through the Epic user interface. Becoming familiar with how to navigate and customize the interface is essential for effectively using Epic in your healthcare practice or organization.

Section 1: Getting Familiar with Epic's User Interface

3.1 Logging In

Before you can start using Epic, you need to log in. Here's how:

Open your web browser and enter the URL provided by your organization for accessing Epic.

Enter your username and password.

Depending on your organization's security policies, you may need to use multi-factor authentication (MFA) for added security.

3.2 Home Screen

Once you're logged in, you'll typically arrive at your home screen. The home screen is your starting point for accessing various Epic modules and functions.

Take a moment to explore the home screen. You'll often find shortcuts to commonly used tools and applications here.

Section 2: Customizing Your Epic Workspace

3.3 Personalizing Your Dashboard

Epic allows you to customize your workspace to make it more efficient for your specific role. Here's how to personalize your dashboard:

Look for options like "Customize" or "Edit Dashboard" on your home screen.

You can usually add or remove widgets, rearrange them, and resize them to suit your preferences.

Common widgets include appointment schedules, patient lists, and task lists.

3.4 Navigating the Epic Menu

The Epic menu is typically located on the left side of the screen. It provides access to different Epic modules and functions. Here's how to navigate it:

Expand and collapse menu sections to find the module you need.

Click on a module to access its features and tools.

Some modules may have sub-menus that further organize their functions.

3.5 Searching for Patients

A crucial part of using Epic is quickly finding patient records. To search for a patient:

Use the search bar at the top of the screen.

You can search by patient name, medical record number, or other identifiers.

Click on the patient's name in the search results to access their record.

Section 3: Customizing Epic for Your Workflow

3.6 Personalization Options

Epic offers various personalization options to tailor the interface to your needs:

User Preferences: Explore the user preferences section to configure default settings for your account, such as your preferred language and display options.

Favorites: You can mark frequently used tools and functions as favorites for easy access.

Order Sets: Depending on your role, you might have the option to create order sets, which are predefined sets of orders you frequently use.

3.7 Epic Training and Resources

Epic often provides training and resources to help users become more proficient with the interface. Check with your organization for access to:

Epic Training Modules: These are usually available online and cover various aspects of using Epic.
Epic User Guides: Detailed guides and documentation can be invaluable resources for learning more about Epic's features.

Section 4: Tips for Efficient Navigation

3.8 Keyboard Shortcuts

Epic often includes keyboard shortcuts to speed up common tasks. These shortcuts can vary depending on your organization's configuration, so it's essential to check with your Epic administrator for a list of available shortcuts.

3.9 Regular Updates

Keep in mind that Epic interfaces may receive updates and enhancements. Staying informed about these changes through your organization's communication channels is crucial to maintaining proficiency.

In the next chapter, we'll explore patient records in Epic, including how to create and manage them efficiently. This knowledge will be essential for healthcare providers and administrators using Epic for patient care and management.

Chapter 4: Patient Records in Epic

In this chapter, we'll delve into the world of patient records within Epic. Understanding how to create, access, and manage patient records is fundamental for healthcare professionals and administrators using Epic for electronic health records (EHR).

Section 1: Creating and Accessing Patient Records

4.1 Patient Registration

To create a patient record in Epic:

Access the "Patient Registration" module from the Epic menu.

Enter the patient's demographic information, including name, date of birth, contact details, and insurance information.

Assign a unique medical record number (MRN) to the patient.

Save the record to create a new patient profile.

4.2 Accessing Patient Records

To access an existing patient record in Epic:

Use the search bar at the top of the screen to search for the patient by name, MRN, or other identifiers.

Click on the patient's name in the search results to open their record.

Section 2: Navigating the Patient Record

4.3 Overview of the Patient Record

Once you've opened a patient's record, you'll find various sections and tabs containing essential information:

Demographics: Basic patient information such as name, date of birth, and contact details.

Clinical Notes: A history of clinical encounters and progress notes.

Medications: A list of current and past medications prescribed to the patient.

Allergies: Information about any known allergies or adverse reactions.

4.4 Navigating Clinical Notes

Clinical notes are a crucial part of the patient record. Here's how to navigate them:

You'll typically find a chronological list of clinical notes, with the most recent note displayed first.

Click on a note to open it and view the details.

You can often filter clinical notes by type, such as progress notes, consultation notes, or discharge summaries.

Section 3: Managing Patient Data

4.5 Adding Clinical Notes

To add a clinical note to a patient's record:

Navigate to the "Clinical Notes" section.

Click on "Add Note" or a similar option.

Complete the note, including details of the encounter, assessment, and plan.

Save the note to add it to the patient's record.

4.6 Medication Management

Epic also allows for efficient medication management:

To prescribe medications, access the "Medications" section of the patient record.

Search for the medication, select the appropriate dose and instructions, and submit the prescription.

Epic often includes built-in drug interaction checking to help prevent medication-related issues.

Section 4: Best Practices for Epic Clinical Documentation

4.7 Documentation Accuracy

Ensure that your clinical notes are accurate, complete, and reflect the patient's condition and treatment accurately.

Use standardized terminology and follow your organization's documentation guidelines.

4.8 Timely Documentation

Document clinical encounters promptly to maintain an up-to-date patient record.

Timely documentation is crucial for continuity of care and legal reasons.

Section 5: Epic Tips and Shortcuts

4.9 Shortcuts and Templates

Explore the use of shortcuts and templates for common clinical documentation to save time and improve consistency.

Templates can be customized to match your specialty and specific documentation needs.

4.10 Alerts and Reminders

Pay attention to alerts and reminders within Epic, as they can prompt you to take necessary actions, such as ordering tests or medications.

Configure your alert preferences to suit your workflow.

In the next chapter, we'll explore clinical documentation in Epic in more detail, including how to efficiently chart and take clinical notes. This knowledge is essential for healthcare providers who use Epic for patient care.

Chapter 5: Clinical Documentation in Epic

In this chapter, we'll dive into the essential aspect of clinical documentation within Epic. Learning how to efficiently chart and take clinical notes is crucial for healthcare providers using Epic for patient care.

Section 1: Efficient Charting and Note Taking

5.1 Types of Clinical Notes
Epic typically supports various types of clinical notes, including:
Progress Notes: Used to document patient encounters, including history, physical examination findings, and assessments.
Consultation Notes: Created when a specialist is consulted for a patient's care.
Procedure Notes: Document details of procedures performed on the patient.

5.2 Navigating Clinical Documentation
To start charting and taking clinical notes:
Access the patient's record and navigate to the "Clinical Notes" section.
Depending on your organization's setup, you may have options like "Create Note" or "Chart Review" to begin documentation.

5.3 Efficient Note Taking
Here are some tips for efficient note taking in Epic:

Use Templates: Epic often provides templates for various note types. Utilize these templates to structure your notes efficiently.

Voice Recognition: Some organizations integrate voice recognition software, allowing you to dictate notes, which can save time.

Copy Forward: If the patient's condition hasn't significantly changed, you can copy forward information from previous notes and update as necessary.

Section 2: Best Practices for Epic Clinical Documentation

5.4 Clarity and Detail
Your notes should be clear, concise, and sufficiently detailed to communicate the patient's condition and your assessment. Include relevant information such as vital signs, allergies, medications, and any changes in the patient's condition.

5.5 Timeliness
Document patient encounters in a timely manner to ensure that the patient's record remains up-to-date and accurate. Timely documentation is essential for continuity of care and legal reasons.

Section 3: Templates and Customization

5.6 Template Usage
Explore the available note templates in Epic, which can help you streamline documentation and ensure that critical elements are included in your notes.

Customize templates to match your specialty and specific documentation needs.

5.7 Customization Options

Depending on your role and organization's setup, you may have the option to customize templates, order sets, and other documentation tools.

Work with your organization's Epic administrator to make necessary customizations that align with your practice's requirements.

Section 4: Epic Tips and Shortcuts

5.8 Shortcuts and SmartPhrases

Epic often includes shortcuts and SmartPhrases, which are predefined text snippets you can insert into your notes. Learn to use these shortcuts to speed up documentation and maintain consistency.

5.9 Documentation Review

Periodically review your clinical documentation for accuracy and completeness.

Consider peer review processes within your organization to enhance documentation quality.

In the next chapter, we'll explore the management of orders and medications in Epic, providing guidance on how to place orders efficiently and ensure medication safety using the system. This knowledge is crucial for healthcare providers who rely on Epic for patient care and management.

Chapter 6: Orders and Medication Management in Epic

In this chapter, we'll delve into the process of managing orders and medications within Epic. Learning how to efficiently place orders and ensure medication safety is essential for healthcare providers using Epic for patient care.

Section 1: Placing Orders in Epic

6.1 Types of Orders

Epic supports various types of orders, including:
Medication Orders: For prescribing and managing medications.
Diagnostic Orders: For requesting and tracking diagnostic tests and procedures.
Treatment Orders: For specifying treatments, therapies, and interventions.

6.2 Placing Orders
To place an order in Epic:
Access the patient's record and navigate to the "Orders" or "Order Entry" section.
Depending on your organization's setup, you may have options like "Place Order" or "Order Entry" to begin the order process.
Select the appropriate order type (e.g., medication, diagnostic, treatment).
Enter the details of the order, including medication name, dosage, route, and frequency.

Review the order for accuracy and completeness before submitting it.

6.3 Order Verification

In many Epic implementations, orders undergo verification by a pharmacist or other healthcare professional before they are carried out. This step ensures that the order is appropriate and safe for the patient.

Section 2: Medication Management and Safety

6.4 Medication Reconciliation

Medication reconciliation is a critical aspect of medication safety:

When admitting a patient, reconcile their current medications with the medications prescribed in Epic to avoid duplication or omissions.

Update medication lists as patients' regimens change.

6.5 Drug Interaction Checking

Epic typically includes built-in drug interaction checking to help prevent medication-related issues:

As you enter a medication order, Epic may provide alerts for potential drug interactions, allergies, or other safety concerns.

Review and resolve these alerts before finalizing the order.

Section 3: Best Practices for Medication Management

6.6 Accurate Medication Documentation

Ensure that medication orders are documented accurately, including dosage, administration route, frequency, and any special instructions.

6.7 Patient Education

Use Epic to document patient education regarding medications, including side effects, dosage instructions, and the importance of compliance.

6.8 Order Review
Periodically review active orders to ensure that they are still clinically appropriate and necessary.

Discontinue orders that are no longer needed.

Section 4: Epic Tips and Shortcuts

6.9 Order Sets
Explore and use order sets, which are predefined groups of orders commonly used for specific conditions or procedures. Order sets can save time and ensure that necessary orders are not overlooked.

6.10 Barcode Medication Administration (BCMA)
If your organization uses BCMA, learn how to scan patient wristbands and medication barcodes to ensure the right patient receives the right medication at the right time.

BCMA enhances medication safety and reduces errors.

In the next chapter, we'll explore Epic's reporting and analytics capabilities, helping you harness the power of data to make informed decisions and improve patient care. This knowledge is valuable for healthcare providers and administrators seeking to leverage data within Epic.

Chapter 7: Epic's Reporting and Analytics

In this chapter, we'll dive into the world of reporting and analytics within Epic. Understanding how to leverage data for decision-making is crucial for healthcare professionals and administrators using Epic to improve patient care and operational efficiency.

Section 1: The Power of Data in Healthcare

7.1 Importance of Data in Healthcare

Data is the lifeblood of healthcare, and Epic provides robust tools to harness its power:

Data-driven decisions can lead to improved patient outcomes, cost savings, and enhanced operational efficiency.

Epic's reporting and analytics capabilities enable you to access, analyze, and visualize data to support your goals.

Section 2: Accessing Data in Epic

7.2 Data Sources

Epic pulls data from various sources, including:

Patient records: Clinical notes, lab results, and vital signs.

Orders and medications: Details of treatments and medications prescribed.

Billing and claims data: Financial information related to patient care.

7.3 Report Types

Epic offers different types of reports to meet various needs:

Standard Reports: Predefined reports that cover common healthcare metrics and KPIs.

Ad Hoc Reports: Customizable reports that allow you to specify the data and criteria you want to analyze.

Section 3: Building Custom Reports

7.4 Creating an Ad Hoc Report

To create a custom report in Epic:

Access the "Reporting" or "Analytics" section from the Epic menu.

Select "Create Report" or a similar option.

Choose the data source, specify criteria, and select the variables you want to include.

Customize the report layout and formatting as needed.

Save or run the report to view the results.

7.5 Visualizing Data

Epic often includes data visualization tools, such as charts and graphs, to help you make sense of the data:

Utilize these tools to present data in a visually engaging and informative manner.

Charts and graphs can make it easier to identify trends and patterns in the data.

Section 4: Realizing the Benefits of Epic Analytics

7.6 Quality Improvement
Analyze clinical data to identify areas for quality improvement and implement evidence-based practices.
Monitor patient outcomes and track progress toward quality goals.

7.7 Financial Management
Use financial reports to manage revenue, track billing and claims, and identify opportunities for cost savings.
Improve reimbursement processes by identifying coding and documentation errors.

7.8 Population Health
Leverage Epic's analytics to assess the health of specific patient populations and target interventions accordingly.
Identify at-risk patients and proactively manage their care to prevent complications.

Section 5: Epic Tips and Shortcuts

7.9 Scheduled Reports
Explore the option to schedule and automate the generation of reports in Epic.

Scheduled reports can save time and ensure that data is regularly updated for analysis.

7.10 Training and Resources

Epic often provides training and resources for users interested in building and analyzing reports.

Take advantage of these resources to enhance your reporting skills.

In the next chapter, we'll explore Epic's role in interoperability, including how to integrate Epic with other healthcare systems and achieve seamless data exchange. This knowledge is essential for healthcare providers and organizations looking to enhance collaboration and data sharing.

Chapter 8: Epic's Role in Interoperability

In this chapter, we'll explore how Epic facilitates interoperability in healthcare. Understanding how to integrate Epic with other healthcare systems and achieve seamless data exchange is crucial for healthcare professionals and administrators seeking to improve collaboration and data sharing.

Section 1: The Importance of Interoperability

8.1 Interoperability in Healthcare
Interoperability refers to the ability of different healthcare systems and applications to exchange and use data seamlessly. Epic plays a significant role in achieving interoperability, and here's why it matters:
Improved care coordination: Interoperability allows different providers and healthcare organizations to share patient information, leading to better-coordinated care.
Reduced errors: Access to a patient's complete health record helps prevent medication errors, duplications, and omissions.
Enhanced patient experience: Patients benefit from a more connected healthcare system, as they don't need to repeatedly provide the same information to different providers.

Section 2: Data Sharing with Epic
8.2 Epic's Approach to Interoperability

Epic follows industry standards and offers several tools and features to support data sharing:

HL7 and FHIR Standards: Epic supports industry-standard data exchange formats like HL7 and FHIR (Fast Healthcare Interoperability Resources) to ensure compatibility with other systems.

Epic Care Everywhere: Epic's Care Everywhere feature enables the exchange of patient records with other healthcare organizations that use Epic.

Interconnectivity: Epic allows for the integration of various data sources, including external laboratories and radiology centers, to bring data into the Epic EHR.

Section 3: Achieving Seamless Data Exchange

8.3 Epic Care Everywhere

Epic Care Everywhere is a critical component of interoperability within the Epic ecosystem:

Learn how to use Care Everywhere to access patient records from other Epic organizations when needed for patient care.

Understand the consent management process to ensure that patient data is shared in compliance with privacy regulations.

8.4 Integrating External Data
Epic often supports interfaces and integration tools to connect with external systems:

Work with your organization's IT department or Epic administrator to set up interfaces with external laboratories, imaging centers, and other healthcare systems.

Ensure that data flow is secure and reliable to maintain data integrity.

Section 4: Realizing the Benefits of Interoperability

8.5 Improved Care Coordination

Interoperability enables healthcare providers to access up-to-date patient information, leading to more informed decisions and better-coordinated care.

Care teams can seamlessly share information, reducing the risk of medical errors and improving patient outcomes.

8.6 Patient Engagement

Patients can access their health records and participate more actively in their care when data is easily accessible across different providers and systems.
Telehealth and remote monitoring are more effective with interoperability, enhancing patient engagement.

Section 5: Epic Tips and Shortcuts
8.7 Epic Support and Resources
Epic often provides training and resources related to interoperability.
Familiarize yourself with Epic's documentation and support

channels to troubleshoot any interoperability issues and maximize data sharing capabilities.

In the next chapter, we'll explore practice management with Epic, including how to streamline administrative processes, appointment scheduling, and billing. This knowledge is essential for healthcare administrators and staff using Epic for practice management tasks.

Chapter 9: Practice Management with Epic

In this chapter, we'll delve into the world of practice management with Epic. Understanding how to streamline administrative processes, appointment scheduling, and billing is essential for healthcare administrators and staff using Epic for practice management tasks.

Section 1: The Role of Practice Management in Healthcare

9.1 Importance of Practice Management
Practice management encompasses a wide range of administrative tasks that ensure the efficient operation of healthcare practices or organizations. Epic offers tools to support these tasks, and here's why it matters:
Improved efficiency: Practice management tools in Epic help streamline administrative workflows, reducing manual tasks and saving time.
Enhanced patient experience: Efficient scheduling, billing, and registration processes lead to a better patient experience.
Financial stability: Effective practice management can optimize revenue collection and reduce billing errors.

Section 2: Streamlining Administrative Processes

9.2 Appointment Scheduling
Epic's appointment scheduling features help you manage patient appointments effectively:

Learn how to schedule, reschedule, and cancel appointments within Epic.

Utilize features like waitlists and overbooking to maximize appointment availability.

9.3 Patient Registration and Check-In

Efficient patient registration and check-in processes are essential:

Use Epic to gather patient demographic information, insurance details, and consent forms.

Streamline the check-in process with electronic forms and digital signatures when possible.

Section 3: Billing and Revenue Cycle Management

9.4 Billing and Claims

Epic's billing and claims management tools are crucial for revenue cycle optimization:

Understand how to generate and submit claims electronically through Epic.

Learn how to review and correct claim denials to ensure timely reimbursement.

9.5 Insurance Verification

Insurance verification is key to accurate billing:

Use Epic to verify patient insurance coverage and eligibility.

Ensure that insurance information is up-to-date to prevent claim denials.

Section 4: Realizing the Benefits of Practice Management in Epic

9.6 Operational Efficiency

Efficient practice management in Epic leads to smoother workflows, reduced administrative overhead, and better staff productivity.

Streamlined processes help practices operate more smoothly and provide a better experience for patients.

9.7 Revenue Maximization

Effective billing and claims management lead to improved revenue collection, reducing financial strain on the practice.

Minimizing claim denials and rejections ensures that the practice is reimbursed promptly and accurately.

Section 5: Epic Tips and Shortcuts

9.8 Epic Training and Resources

Epic often provides training and resources for practice management tasks.

Familiarize yourself with Epic's documentation, attend training sessions, and seek support from your organization's

Epic administrator to optimize practice management processes.

In the next chapter, we'll explore workflow optimization in Epic, helping you design efficient workflows and customize Epic to meet your specific needs. This knowledge is valuable for healthcare administrators and staff seeking to maximize the benefits of Epic for their practice or organization.

Chapter 10: Workflow Optimization in Epic

In this chapter, we'll explore the art of workflow optimization in Epic. Learning how to design efficient workflows and customize Epic to meet your specific needs is crucial for healthcare administrators and staff seeking to maximize the benefits of the system.

Section 1: The Importance of Workflow Optimization

10.1 Efficiency in Healthcare

Efficient workflows are essential in healthcare for several reasons:

Reducing administrative burden: Streamlined processes allow healthcare providers to focus on patient care rather than paperwork.

Enhanced patient experience: Efficient workflows mean shorter wait times and smoother interactions for patients.

Cost savings: Improved efficiency can lead to cost savings for healthcare organizations.

Section 2: Designing Efficient Workflows

10.2 Workflow Analysis
Before you can optimize workflows, you need to understand them:

Conduct a workflow analysis to identify current processes, pain points, and areas for improvement.

Gather input from staff members who are directly involved in the workflows to gain valuable insights.

10.3 Redesigning Workflows

Once you've analyzed the existing workflows, it's time to redesign them:

Identify opportunities to automate manual tasks using Epic's features.

Streamline the flow of information and tasks to minimize handoffs and delays.

Section 3: Customizing Epic for Your Workflow

10.4 Customization Options

Epic is highly customizable to adapt to your specific workflows:

Explore the customization options available in your Epic implementation.

Work with your organization's Epic administrator or IT department to make necessary adjustments.

10.5 Order Sets and Templates

Utilize order sets and templates to further streamline workflows:

Create custom order sets for common procedures or diagnoses to save time when ordering tests or treatments.

Customize templates for clinical documentation to ensure consistency and efficiency.

Section 4: Realizing the Benefits of Workflow Optimization

10.6 Improved Efficiency

Efficient workflows lead to improved efficiency in healthcare settings:

Reduced wait times for patients.

Faster clinical decision-making.

More time for patient care and less time on administrative tasks.

10.7 Better Patient Experience

Patients benefit from optimized workflows:
Shorter wait times for appointments.

Less paperwork and redundant data entry.

Enhanced communication between healthcare providers.

Section 5: Epic Tips and Shortcuts
10.8 User Training
Ensure that staff members are properly trained in using Epic's features and customizations related to your workflow.

Continuous training and regular updates are crucial to maximizing the benefits of workflow optimization.

10.9 Continuous Improvement

Workflow optimization is an ongoing process. Regularly review and refine your workflows to adapt to changing needs and technologies.

In the next chapter, we'll explore Epic's security and compliance features, helping you protect patient data and ensure that your organization remains compliant with healthcare regulations. This knowledge is vital for healthcare administrators and staff responsible for data security and compliance in Epic.

Chapter 11: Security and Compliance in Epic

In this chapter, we'll delve into the realm of security and compliance within Epic. Understanding how to protect patient data and ensure your organization complies with healthcare regulations is vital for healthcare administrators and staff responsible for data security and compliance in Epic.

Section 1: The Importance of Security and Compliance

11.1 Data Security in Healthcare

Data security is a top priority in healthcare for several reasons:
Protecting patient privacy: Healthcare organizations must safeguard patient information to maintain trust and comply with legal requirements.
Preventing data breaches: Security measures help prevent unauthorized access to sensitive data.
Compliance with regulations: Healthcare is subject to various regulations like HIPAA (Health Insurance Portability and Accountability Act) that impose strict data security requirements.

Section 2: Epic's Security Features
11.2 User Authentication
Epic employs robust user authentication methods to ensure only authorized personnel access patient data:

Learn about Epic's login security measures, which may include strong password requirements and multi-factor authentication (MFA).

Follow best practices for password management to maintain account security.

11.3 Role-Based Access Control (RBAC)

Epic often implements RBAC to control access to different parts of the system:

Understand how RBAC works and how roles and permissions are assigned within Epic.

Ensure that users have the appropriate access rights based on their roles and responsibilities.

Section 3: Compliance with Regulations

11.4 HIPAA Compliance

HIPAA sets the standard for protecting sensitive patient data:

Familiarize yourself with HIPAA regulations, including the Privacy Rule, Security Rule, and Breach Notification Rule.

Ensure that your organization's use of Epic aligns with HIPAA requirements, including patient consent and data encryption.

11.5 Other Regulatory Requirements

Depending on your location and practice, other regulations may apply:

Stay informed about relevant local, state, and international data protection laws, such as GDPR (General Data Protection Regulation) in the European Union.

Work with legal and compliance teams to ensure Epic usage aligns with all applicable regulations.

Section 4: Data Encryption and Auditing

11.6 Data Encryption
Epic often uses encryption to protect data both at rest and in transit:
Understand how encryption works within Epic, including secure communication protocols and data storage practices. Ensure that encryption is enabled and properly configured in your Epic environment.

11.7 Auditing and Monitoring
Epic includes auditing and monitoring features to track user activities and potential security incidents:
Review audit logs regularly to identify and respond to any unusual or suspicious activities.
Establish incident response procedures to address security breaches promptly.

Section 5: Realizing the Benefits of Security and Compliance

11.8 Patient Trust
Effective security and compliance measures build patient

trust by assuring them that their data is being handled responsibly and securely.

11.9 Legal and Financial Protection

Compliance with regulations and robust security measures protect your organization from legal and financial consequences of data breaches and non-compliance.

Section 6: Epic Tips and Shortcuts

11.10 Ongoing Training and Awareness

Regularly train staff members on security and compliance best practices, and keep them informed about any policy changes or updates.

Foster a culture of security awareness within your organization.

In the next chapter, we'll explore disaster recovery and data backup strategies in Epic, helping you ensure the continuity of patient care and data availability in the face of unexpected events. This knowledge is critical for healthcare administrators and IT staff responsible for data protection and business continuity in Epic.

Chapter 12: Disaster Recovery and Data Backup in Epic

In this chapter, we'll explore the crucial aspects of disaster recovery and data backup strategies within Epic. Understanding how to safeguard patient data, ensure business continuity, and recover from unexpected events is essential for healthcare administrators and IT staff responsible for data protection and system resilience in Epic.

Section 1: The Importance of Disaster Recovery and Data Backup

12.1 Data Protection and Business Continuity
Disaster recovery and data backup are essential for healthcare organizations for several reasons:
Protecting patient data: Ensuring that patient information remains safe and accessible, even in the event of disasters or system failures.
Business continuity: Maintaining healthcare operations during and after unexpected events, such as natural disasters, cyberattacks, or hardware failures.

Section 2: Data Backup in Epic

12.2 Backup Strategies
Epic typically employs various backup strategies to protect data:

Learn about the types of backups used, including full backups, incremental backups, and differential backups.

Understand the backup frequency and retention policies in place within your organization.

12.3 Data Retention

Epic also often implements data retention policies:

Familiarize yourself with how long different types of data are retained in backups and what happens when data reaches the end of its retention period.

Ensure compliance with legal and regulatory requirements regarding data retention.

Section 3: Disaster Recovery Planning

12.4 Disaster Recovery Plans

Disaster recovery plans are essential to quickly recover from unexpected events:

Work with your organization's IT team to develop a comprehensive disaster recovery plan that outlines roles, responsibilities, and procedures to follow during and after a disaster.

Consider scenarios such as data center failures, natural disasters, and cybersecurity incidents when creating your plan.

12.5 Testing and Drills

Regular testing and drills are critical for disaster recovery preparedness:

Conduct disaster recovery exercises to ensure that staff members are familiar with the plan and can execute it effectively.

Identify and address any weaknesses or gaps in the plan through testing.

Section 4: Realizing the Benefits of Disaster Recovery and Data Backup

12.6 Data Resilience

Robust disaster recovery and data backup strategies ensure that patient data remains available and secure, even in the face of unexpected events.

12.7 Business Continuity

Effective disaster recovery planning and data backup measures minimize downtime, allowing healthcare organizations to continue providing critical services.

Section 5: Epic Tips and Shortcuts

12.8 Offsite Backup

Consider storing backups offsite to protect against physical disasters that may affect the primary data center.

Implement secure data transfer protocols when sending backups offsite to ensure data integrity and confidentiality.

12.9 Regular Review and Updates

Periodically review and update your disaster recovery plan and backup strategies to account for changes in technology, regulations, and the organization's needs.

In the next chapter, we'll explore Epic's reporting and analytics capabilities in more detail, helping you harness the power of data for clinical and operational insights. This knowledge is valuable for healthcare administrators and analysts seeking to leverage data within Epic.

Chapter 13: Advanced Reporting and Analytics in Epic

In this chapter, we'll dive deeper into Epic's reporting and analytics capabilities, focusing on advanced techniques and features. Understanding how to harness the power of data for clinical and operational insights is essential for healthcare administrators, analysts, and advanced users looking to maximize the benefits of Epic's reporting and analytics tools.

Section 1: Advanced Reporting Techniques

13.1 Custom Reports and Dashboards

Epic's advanced reporting allows for the creation of custom reports and dashboards tailored to your specific needs:

Explore the tools for designing custom reports and dashboards within Epic's reporting module.

Learn how to select and organize key performance indicators (KPIs) that provide actionable insights.

13.2 Data Integration

Integrating data from multiple sources can provide a comprehensive view of healthcare operations:

Understand how to integrate external data sources, such as financial data, patient satisfaction surveys, and population health data, into your Epic reports and dashboards.

Use data transformation and cleansing techniques to ensure data quality and accuracy.

Section 2: Advanced Analytics

13.3 Predictive Analytics

Predictive analytics can help forecast patient outcomes and resource needs:

Explore the use of predictive models within Epic to identify at-risk patients and allocate resources effectively.

Learn how to create and validate predictive models using historical patient data.

13.4 Machine Learning

Epic may offer machine learning capabilities for advanced analytics:
Understand how to apply machine learning algorithms to tasks like readmission prediction, disease diagnosis, and patient risk stratification.

Collaborate with data scientists or analysts to develop and deploy machine learning models within Epic.

Section 3: Operational Insights

13.5 Operational Efficiency

Epic's reporting and analytics can be leveraged to improve operational efficiency:

Analyze data related to patient flow, appointment scheduling, and resource allocation to identify areas for optimization. Use data-driven insights to streamline workflows and reduce operational costs.

13.6 Resource Allocation
Efficient resource allocation is crucial for delivering quality care:
Utilize Epic's analytics to assess resource utilization, including staffing levels, equipment, and facilities.
Optimize resource allocation based on patient demand and clinical need.

Section 4: Realizing the Benefits of Advanced Reporting and Analytics

13.7 Informed Decision-Making
Advanced reporting and analytics provide decision-makers with data-driven insights that lead to more informed decisions and improved patient care.

13.8 Continuous Improvement
Regularly review and refine your reporting and analytics strategies to adapt to evolving healthcare needs and technology advancements.

Section 5: Epic Tips and Shortcuts
13.9 Epic Support and Training
Take advantage of Epic's advanced training and support resources for reporting and analytics.

Collaborate with Epic experts and data analysts to stay up-to-date with best practices and advanced techniques.

In the next chapter, we'll explore interoperability in Epic in greater detail, including how to exchange data with external healthcare systems, organizations, and platforms. This knowledge is valuable for healthcare administrators and IT staff seeking to enhance collaboration and data sharing using Epic.

Chapter 14: Interoperability and Data Exchange in Epic

In this chapter, we'll delve deeper into the world of interoperability in Epic. Understanding how to exchange data with external healthcare systems, organizations, and platforms is crucial for healthcare administrators, IT staff, and clinicians seeking to enhance collaboration and data sharing using Epic.

Section 1: Data Exchange Standards

14.1 HL7 and FHIR

Epic supports industry-standard data exchange formats, including HL7 (Health Level Seven) and FHIR (Fast Healthcare Interoperability Resources):

Learn how to use these standards to facilitate data exchange between Epic and external systems.

Understand the role of HL7 and FHIR in ensuring interoperability across the healthcare ecosystem.

14.2 Integration Engines

Integration engines play a vital role in data exchange:

Explore the use of integration engines to map, transform, and route data between Epic and external systems.

Understand the importance of message routing and data transformation in achieving seamless interoperability.

Section 2: HIEs and Data Sharing Networks

14.3 Health Information Exchanges (HIEs)

HIEs enable the sharing of patient data across multiple healthcare organizations:

Learn how to connect Epic with HIEs to access a broader network of patient information.
Understand the benefits of HIEs, such as improved care coordination and access to patient records from other healthcare providers.

14.4 Data Sharing Networks

Data sharing networks allow for collaborative care and data exchange:
Explore how Epic facilitates data sharing within these networks, which may include referral networks and regional health information organizations (RHIOs).
Understand the role of data sharing networks in improving patient care and reducing duplication of tests and treatments.

Section 3: External Data Integration
14.5 Lab and Imaging Systems
Epic often integrates with external laboratory and imaging systems:

Learn how to establish and maintain connections with these systems to ensure seamless data exchange for test results and images.

Understand the benefits of real-time access to laboratory and imaging data within Epic.

14.6 Pharmacy Systems

Pharmacy systems integration is essential for medication management:

Explore the integration of Epic with pharmacy systems to facilitate electronic prescribing and medication reconciliation.

Ensure accurate and up-to-date medication information within the EHR.

Section 4: Realizing the Benefits of Interoperability

14.7 Enhanced Care Coordination

Interoperability enables healthcare providers to access comprehensive patient information, leading to better-coordinated care and improved patient outcomes.

14.8 Efficiency and Cost Savings

By reducing manual data entry and improving access to external data, interoperability enhances efficiency and can lead to cost savings for healthcare organizations.

Section 5: Epic Tips and Shortcuts

14.9 Epic's Interoperability Toolkit

Familiarize yourself with Epic's interoperability toolkit and resources, which can help streamline the integration process.

Stay informed about updates and enhancements to Epic's interoperability features to take full advantage of their capabilities.

In the next chapter, we'll explore Epic's telehealth capabilities, including how to leverage the platform for virtual patient care and remote consultations. This knowledge is valuable for healthcare providers and organizations seeking to expand their telehealth services using Epic.

Chapter 15: Telehealth with Epic

In this chapter, we'll dive into Epic's telehealth capabilities, focusing on how to leverage the platform for virtual patient care and remote consultations. Understanding telehealth in Epic is crucial for healthcare providers and organizations looking to expand their telehealth services and provide convenient care options to patients.

Section 1: The Importance of Telehealth

15.1 Telehealth in Healthcare
Telehealth has become an essential component of healthcare for various reasons:
Expanding access: Telehealth allows patients to receive care remotely, overcoming geographical barriers.
Convenience: Virtual consultations provide patients with more flexible options for receiving medical advice and treatment.
Continuity of care: Telehealth ensures that patients can access care even during emergencies or situations that limit in-person visits.

Section 2: Telehealth Setup in Epic

15.2 Telehealth Features in Epic

Epic typically offers a range of telehealth features to support remote patient care:

Explore Epic's telehealth capabilities, including videoconferencing, secure messaging, and virtual visit scheduling.

Familiarize yourself with the specific telehealth tools and modules available in your organization's Epic implementation.

15.3 Integration with Scheduling

Epic often integrates telehealth with appointment scheduling:

Learn how to schedule virtual appointments within Epic, ensuring that patients and providers have access to the necessary information for virtual visits.

Understand the process for rescheduling or canceling virtual appointments.

Section 3: Conducting Virtual Visits

15.4 Preparing for Virtual Visits

Successful virtual visits require preparation:

Ensure that both patients and providers have the required hardware (computer, webcam, microphone) and a stable internet connection.

Communicate instructions to patients for accessing the virtual visit platform within Epic.

15.5 Conducting the Virtual Visit

During the virtual visit:

Use Epic's videoconferencing tools to conduct the consultation and provide medical advice.

Document the virtual visit within the patient's EHR, including assessments, prescriptions, and recommendations.

Section 4: Telehealth Benefits and Considerations

15.6 Patient Experience

Telehealth enhances the patient experience by providing a convenient and accessible way to receive medical care.

Patients appreciate the flexibility and reduced travel associated with virtual visits.

15.7 Provider Efficiency

Telehealth can improve provider efficiency by reducing wait times and allowing for more flexible scheduling.

Providers can see patients from remote locations, expanding their reach.

15.8 Legal and Regulatory Considerations

Familiarize yourself with telehealth regulations and reimbursement policies specific to your region and practice.

Ensure compliance with privacy and security regulations (e.g., HIPAA) when conducting virtual visits.

Section 5: Epic Tips and Shortcuts

15.9 Epic Telehealth Training

Take advantage of Epic's telehealth training resources and support to become proficient in using telehealth features.

Keep up-to-date with Epic's telehealth updates and enhancements to maximize the benefits of the platform.

With this knowledge, you can effectively incorporate telehealth into your healthcare practice, providing convenient and accessible care options to your patients using Epic.

Made in United States
Orlando, FL
29 May 2025

61653668R10033